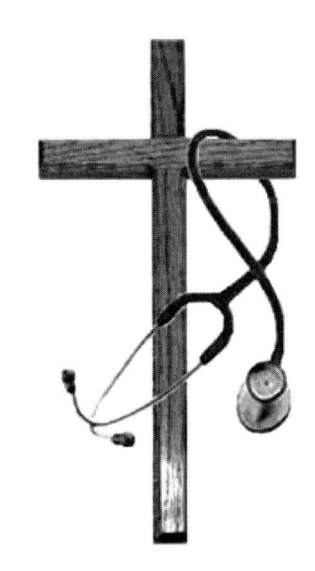

MEDICINE FOR NURSES

© Copyright 2005 Jenny Morris.

All rights reserved. No part of this publication may be reproduced, stored in a retrieval system, or transmitted, in any form or by any means, electronic, mechanical, photocopying, recording, or otherwise, without the written prior permission of the author.

All scripture is from the King James Version of the Bible.
Editor: Belinda Looney

Note for Librarians: a cataloguing record for this book that includes Dewey Decimal Classification and US Library of Congress numbers is available from the Library and Archives of Canada. The complete cataloguing record can be obtained from their online database at:
www.collectionscanada.ca/amicus/index-e.html
ISBN 1-4120-5008-1

TRAFFORD
PUBLISHING

Offices in Canada, USA, Ireland and UK

This book was published *on-demand* in cooperation with Trafford Publishing. On-demand publishing is a unique process and service of making a book available for retail sale to the public taking advantage of on-demand manufacturing and Internet marketing. On-demand publishing includes promotions, retail sales, manufacturing, order fulfilment, accounting and collecting royalties on behalf of the author.

Book sales for North America and international:
Trafford Publishing, 6E–2333 Government St.,
Victoria, BC v8t 4p4 CANADA
phone 250 383 6864 (toll-free 1 888 232 4444)
fax 250 383 6804; email to orders@trafford.com

Book sales in Europe:
Trafford Publishing (uk) Ltd., Enterprise House, Wistaston Road Business Centre,
Wistaston Road, Crewe, Cheshire cw2 7rp UNITED KINGDOM
phone 01270 251 396 (local rate 0845 230 9601)
facsimile 01270 254 983; orders.uk@trafford.com

Order online at:
trafford.com/04-2816

10 9 8 7 6 5 4 3 2

Goals

There are several goals that I have for this little book of devotions. First and foremost, I want all caregivers that read it to be assured that the Lord is here to help them in whatever need they may have. He is a personal God who knows all of us individually, and if we will allow Him, He will be Lord of our lives. Second, my goal is to help nurses and other healthcare professionals to see how important they are to the service of the Lord. It is through our hands and words that He often ministers to His people who are sick.

Dedication

I love nursing with all my heart and am very proud to be in the nursing profession. But more important to me than being a nurse, or even a mother, a wife or a grandmother is to be a Christian! I dedicate this book to the wonderful lady who helped me come to the saving knowledge of Jesus Christ, Camilla L. Roden, better known at our church as Sister Nell.

Contents

A Special Acknowledgement	9
A Special Thanks	11
Introduction: Why I Became a Nurse	13
A Broken Heart	17
A Merry Heart	19
Bonding	21
But Then…	23
Changes	25
Confidence	27
Five Rights	29
Gave Blood-Gave Life	31
Good Report	33
Guardian Angel	35
A Nurse's Prayer (Poem)	37
Helping Hands	39
If You Don't Use It, You Lose It	41
Is It Really More Blessed to Give Than to Receive?	43
Life Is in the Blood	45

Little Ailments	47
Expectations (Poem)	49
Making It Through	51
Many Members	53
Marrow To Thy Bones	55
Mind Set	57
Mission Statement	59
No Procedure Is Small…	61
Nurses' Appreciation Week	63
Personal God	65
Puzzles, Pieces, and Pictures	67
Rejoicing and Weeping	69
Specialty Areas	71
The Cure	73
The Good Samaritan	75
The Great Physician	77
Thank God for the Blood	79
Wages	81
Epilogue: Counting the Cost	83
My Saviour (Poem)	89
About the Author	91

A Special Acknowledgement

I have been a Christian for over twenty years, and although there have been many times when I have been discouraged, I have never once considered turning back. During those times of discouragement or whenever I felt like I was down in the valley, it was always the preached Word that brought me victory. For that, I am eternally grateful to the two great Pastors in my life, Rev. Bob McCool, Sr. and Rev. Bobby McCool, Jr. The gross majority of any spiritual insight in this little book came from listening to my Pastors, as they would preach this wonderful message of truth! Thank you, Pastors, for giving me a love for the preached Word and for teaching me "The Purpose is Souls!"

A Special Thanks

There have been many people who have helped me with this special project. I send many thanks to the friends, family, and co-workers who read my little devotions. They gave me great feedback, and their opinions were greatly appreciated! I am sincerely grateful for the love and support I have been given by my husband, Bobby, and my two daughters, Holli and Jennifer. Also, I am very thankful to my sisters, Susan and Belinda. Susan spent many hours checking my scripture references and making sure I had them correctly quoted. She is an inspiration to all that know her and is one of my greatest encouragers! Belinda has an awesome gift for writing poetry, and she was gracious enough to allow me to share two poems with you. She is a Registered Nurse, and only her love for God outshines her love for nursing! Belinda, also, generously agreed to be my editor. Last, but not least, thanks to my Dad, John W. Grigsby. He is a great man and, fortunately, taught me not to be afraid of a hard day's work!

Jenny

Introduction: Why I Became a Nurse

Thirty-two patients! Just my luck I have to charge today. That means 32 assessments, 14 piggybacks, and 7 IV pushes. Of course, there's lab to be called, charts to be checked, and doctors to be notified, and all in a timely manner! By the end of my 12-hour, shift I am often worn out. More days than not I've asked myself, "Why did you become a nurse?" After much deliberation, the answer is actually very easy. I've always wanted to have a servant's heart, and being a nurse gives me a perfect opportunity to serve my fellow man.

Our patients have a variety of needs: physical, financial, and spiritual just to name a few. Physical needs are usually the first needs to be met. It is very rewarding to see an admission WBC to drop from 22 to 8 during a patient's hospital visit. To observe temps go down from 102 degrees to 98 and know that you have been a part of the healing process is remarkable!

Being a patient's advocate also means intervening when there are financial needs. Our society today has many people that are without insurance, have a very low income, or just unable to obtain meds or supplies needed to help them cope with the disease process. A call to our social worker or discharge planner puts into motion a plan to help ease the financial burden on our patients.

Being a Christian, my greatest personal reward comes from helping meet my patient's spiritual needs! I remember once I was working on a med/surg floor, and there was a precious lady with terminal cancer. She was AAOX3, but we all knew she was very close to dying. She knew it as well. We would often enter her room and find her praying or praising God. One afternoon several of our staff members went to her room and asked her if she would like for us to pray with her. There were several family members in her room, and one could see the look of appreciation and gratitude on their faces. A few weeks later when I read the obituary, I thought to myself, "What a comfort for her family to know that their mother had caregivers that would take time to care for even her spiritual needs."

A servant's heart! Yes, that's why I became a nurse.

Jenny Morris, RN

MEDICINE FOR NURSES

Short daily devotions taking a nursing
concept and applying a Biblical principle

Jenny Morris, RN

A Broken Heart

Isaiah 61:1–2 **The spirit of the Lord God is upon me; because the Lord hath anointed me to preach good tidings unto the meek; he hath sent me to bind up the broken-hearted, to proclaim liberty to the captives, and the opening of the prison to them that are bound; . . . to comfort all that mourn;**

Coronary artery disease, pericarditis, dysrhythmias, angina; Heart disease, as we know, is the leading cause of death in America today. Fortunately, with proper diet, the right medication, and exercise, many people with these conditions can continue to live productive fulfilling lives. Cardiologists and heart surgeons are greatly admired for their skill and expertise in caring for the diseased heart. But there is one condition that most of us have had at sometime in our lives that a cardiologist or heart surgeon could not help us with at all. It was when we suffered from a "broken heart." It may have been from a failed relationship, the death of a loved one, or severe disappointment in someone. No matter what the cause, a broken heart is one of the hardest things to get over. But, thank God, we have a Savior who specializes in mending broken hearts! God sees how your heart is bleeding from wounds (hurts) of the past. He sees how it has been broken. He loves you so much, and if you let Him, He will heal your broken heart. Whatever has caused that great pain in your life, give it to the Lord and let Him help you.

My prayer for you today: Dear Lord, I know from experience that You can heal a broken heart! I pray that You bring peace, joy, and laughter into the lives of those that are suffering at this time. Be the Comforter to them and comfort them in a way that only You can. Heal their broken hearts when they feel it is broken into a million pieces. But before You bind it back, take out anything not like You. Fill it with peace, love, joy, and happiness.

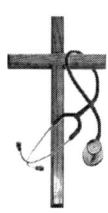

Assignment for the day: Think of a few people that you know who have recently been hurt and say a special prayer for them. If possible, send them a little card of encouragement.

NOTES:

A Merry Heart

Proverbs 17:22 A merry heart doeth good like a medicine: …

Do you ever have one those days when you just get up in the morning feeling wonderful? Maybe it is the memories of the night before, the excitement of special plans for later in the week, or for some other unknown reason you just feel all happy inside! You begin your shift, and it does not matter that you have three patients more than the other nurses. ER calls for a room, and you find out that you're getting that "frequent flyer" that gets on everybody's nerves, and it doesn't dampen your spirit at all! You make your rounds, see all of your patients, and that happy feeling just stays with you all day long. As you make your last check on your patients, it dawns on you," I sure had some good patients today. Yeah, they were sick. But on those last rounds everyone of them was smiling and telling me to have a good day." Did you know that the Bible says, "A merry heart doeth good like a medicine"? When I have read this in the past, I understood it as a merry heart doeth good like a medicine to that individual, and I know that it does. But now as a caregiver, I wonder if, when I have a merry heart, is it possible for it to overflow and affect my patients as a medicine does for them? I think it possibly does! I know it sure can't hurt them. It would be great if I could go to work every day with a "merry heart" and be on top of the world all day long! Realistically, however, those days are few and far between. But still, I can surely enjoy them when they do come!

My prayer for you today: Dear Lord, I pray that You bless all caregivers today. Let them begin their shift with the joy and happiness that comes from knowing

You. Help them to have a merry heart today, and may their joy overflow to their patients!

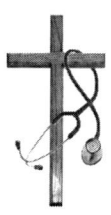

Assignment for the day: Think of two occasions or events in your life that always make you smile when you remember them. Try to keep these thoughts on your mind and throughout the day, if possible, share them with someone. I'm sure it will make you smile, as well!

NOTES:

Bonding

Romans 12:10   Be ye kindly affectioned one to another with brotherly love; in honour preferring one another;

OB nurses will tell you that whenever possible a newborn is placed in his mother's arms within minutes of being born. In fact, over the last few years the "birthing process" has changed dramatically to enhance the bonding period between mother and baby. To develop a sense of trust, the newborn needs to be held close and feel that he is loved. We all remember studying Erikson's eight stages of life, the first being Trust verses Mistrust. Whether it is by the natural parents, adoptive parents, or foster parents, it is vital for the newborn to develop a bond or attachment with those giving care to him. There is much literature available to parents on the importance of bonding with their baby. Unfortunately, when the bonding process does not take place for the newborn, failure to thrive may develop. As we know, this can mean malnutrition with severe complications including death.

Jesus often compared the church to a mother. Spiritually, a new convert is like a newborn baby! Just as infants need a mother to bond with, new converts need a mother (the church) to bond with. The Apostle Paul wrote that a new Christian must be fed milk before he is given meat. He will make many mistakes in learning to live the Christian life. Hopefully, he will have a mother (church) there to help him and to let him know he is loved. Like the loving mother picks up her little toddler when he falls, the church picks up the new converts when they fall. If the bonding process does not take place for the new convert, he, like the newborn, may develop "spiritual" failure to thrive. He may develop spiritual malnutrition. That's why, just as LOVE helps newborns to develop into trusting secure individuals, it is LOVE that helps new converts to develop into strong productive Christians!

My prayer for you today: Dear Lord, I pray that You bless all nurses today. Let love abound in their lives. Because love is what bonds the newborn with his mother and bonds the new convert with the church, I pray that You wrap Your arms around all caregivers and saturate them with Your love.

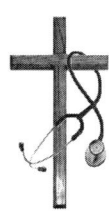

Assignment for the day: Call someone (spouse, children, parents, brothers, or sisters) and tell them that you love them.

NOTES:

But Then...

Ephesians 5:16 Redeeming the time, . . .

Have you ever ended your shift wondering if you had given your patients all the care they needed and deserved? As caregivers, we have all had those days when we barely make it in a patient's room before another patient is calling for something. Often we wonder where the time is going to come from to get all of these assessments, med passes, and treatments done! Something as simple as instilling eye drops can feel like it takes forever when you are in a rush. Whether it is staffing shortage, high acuity of patients, or one of a million other reasons; we have all, no doubt, felt we have fallen short on some days! **But then**, there are days that you leave work feeling so rewarded and fulfilled with your nursing career! You were able to talk with that frightened patient and actually listen to all of his concerns. You were able to sit down with that new diabetic and tell him all about diabetes. You gave him perfect instructions for insulin injections and he was able to return demonstration! As far as eye drops, you were able to sit there and wait the whole-required time between instillations. You know you instilled them perfectly in the conjunctiva! You left work thinking, " Isn't nursing great?"

Isn't that how it is with our prayer life? Some days we get up with only minutes before we have to leave for work. Other days there is so much housework to do you feel like you have to tackle it before you do anything else! The phone starts ringing before you get out of bed and doesn't stop all morning long. You only have one day off, and you have so much to do that you have to get started as soon as you get up! You barely take time to say a simple prayer before you start your hectic day. **But then**, there are those days when you actually get up when the alarm clock goes off.

You have time to drink a cup of coffee, read your Bible, and take time to talk to the Lord before you even start your day! You get to pray for those special people in your life and for the needs of others. I have found it makes all the difference in the world in how my day goes if I can start it off by talking to the Lord!

My prayer for you today: Dear Lord, I pray that You help all caregivers today as they prepare for their busy schedule. Bless them with a few precious minutes to spend praying and reading Your Word before their day begins.

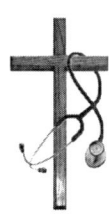

Assignment for the day: When you get to work today before you get out of your vehicle, take a few moments and ask the Lord to protect you (from needle sticks, etc.) and to protect your patients (from med errors, etc).

NOTES:

Changes

II Corinthians 5:17   **Therefore if any man be in Christ, he is a new creature: old things are passed away; behold all things are become new.**

Working in a nursing home/rehab center can be very enlightening! Although some of the residents are fairly young, the majority of them are in their eighties and nineties. There are even a few that are over a hundred! As I give care to them, I often wonder, "What kind of lives did they live when they were younger?" I am almost sure many were young athletes in their day! Most were mothers and fathers that took care of their little babies. We even have retired healthcare professionals. I look at how "Time" has not been very good to them and has caused many changes in their lives. It replaced their smooth skin with wrinkles, and it has robbed them of numerous things. Many have lost their ability to walk by themselves safely, and for others their capability to feed themselves. As healthcare professionals, we recognize that the changes made by time can even rob them of their dignity and self-esteem. There is a saying "Time waits on no man." I suppose this is true. Fortunately, unlike Time, when the Lord saves us, we are changed for the better! I have occasionally sat in church and wondered what kind of lives many had before meeting God! Some of us were almost certainly so far in sin and never dreamed of getting out! Most, however, were probably just good people who had not come to the saving knowledge of Jesus Christ. Only each of us truly knows how the Lord changed us when He saved us! I am so thankful that when He saves us, He doesn't look at what we are, but He looks at what we can be! When the Lord saves us, we get back many things that have been taken. Whether it is our self-esteem, the love of our family, or our joy and peace that is restored, we are blessed to have been "changed" by the Lord!

My prayer for you today: Dear Lord, I pray for all nurses today that may need to have something restored in their lives. Whether it is health, self-esteem, joy, or any other need, I pray that You will intervene and return what may have been taken from them over the years.

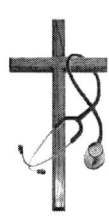

Assignment for the day: Think of one area in your life that has been greatly improved or "changed" by the Lord's help. Take a few minutes and thank Him for it.

NOTES:

Confidence

1 John 5:14–15 **And this is the confidence that we have in him, that, if we ask any thing according to his will, he heareth us: And if we know that he hear us, whatsoever we ask, we know that we have the petitions that we desired of him.**

I remember when I first got out of nursing school and was working as an LPN. I was really nervous about suctioning somebody with a trach. I knew the procedure, I knew what I needed to take with me, and I knew the precautions to take. I just felt insecure in my abilities to do the procedure. Fortunately, I had the best charge nurse; her name was Gail. Every time I needed to suction this patient I would ask her just to go down to the room with me to make sure I was doing it right! Finally one day she said, "Jenny, just go on down there. I'm not going with you because I know you can do it." Sure enough, I suctioned the man without any problems. She gave me the confidence that I needed to realize that I could do the procedure myself. Gail doesn't know it, but I know that she did go down there and stand outside of the door just in case I needed her!

Likewise, as a Christian, there have been many times when I have felt insecure in my ability to pray effectively for others. There are many people with very serious needs, and some of them do not even know God! They do not know Him as the Way Maker, the Peace Speaker, or the Deliverer. Someone has to intervene and go to God in prayer for them. Again, we know the procedure. Pray about it, believe God for the answer, and thank Him for it. But still, when you think about people's needs and the importance of really praying and intervening for others, it can be really frightening. I must confess, there have been many times when I have prayed for someone, and I have wondered if my prayer got through. Thankfully, I have learned, through the preached Word, to take authority and to believe that God will answer my prayers! Learning to put our confidence in God and His Word is one of the greatest realizations we can have!

My prayer for you today: Dear Lord, I pray for all today that may be struggling with insecurities and fears. Whether it is on the job or in their personal lives, I ask that You remind them that they can have confidence in You and Your Word.

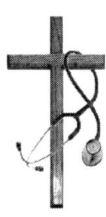

Assignment for the day: If you have co-workers that are new nurses, take a few minutes to encourage them. Maybe you can even share a few tips with them to make their jobs easier.

NOTES:

Five Rights

Romans 3:23   For all have sinned, and come short of the glory of God;

When I was a waitress and made a mistake, it meant someone got meatloaf instead of roast beef or a Coke instead of a Dr. Pepper. When I was a cashier and made a mistake, it meant someone got a little extra (or less) change back than he was due. But as a nurse, I realize that if I make a mistake it can be harmful, even life threatening to my patients. We all know the "5 Rights" for administering medications, and fortunately we have prevented many med errors by checking them before giving our patients their meds. However, many of us have felt that "chill go down our spine" when we realized we had just made a med error! I remember one time I gave Demerol IM to a patient and it was ordered PO. Another time I gave a med that was due QOD on a day that it wasn't due. Gratefully, neither time the patients were harmed. Although we try our very best to be conscientious, we are human and mistakes do happen. We have a protocol to follow when this occurs, and then we must go about doing our jobs to the best of our ability!

Regrettably, I have made many "mistakes" as a Christian. Though they were unintentional, they surely have caused pain or heartache to others. In fact, I have often wandered who pays the price when I fail God? Who did not get witnessed to about His saving power? Who needed encouragement and did not receive it because I was having a bad day? Who was in desperate need of prayer and needed someone to intervene for them? Thankfully, I have found there are certain "Rights" that I can pray for daily to help me from making so many mistakes. When I start my day by asking the Lord to help me to have a "Right Heart, a Right Spirit, a Right Attitude, and to do Right because it's Right to do Right," it seems I have a much better day. I am so thankful the Lord has given us a "protocol" to follow when we make mistakes and is so loving and so just to forgive us!

My prayer for you today: Dear Lord, thank You for being so awesome and so forgiving to us when we make mistakes and fail You. I pray for all caregivers today that You help them in every area of their lives. I pray while on the job today You let them know when they need to do "one more check" on that med they are about to administer. Protect them and protect their patients, in Jesus name we pray.

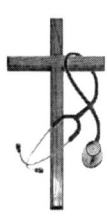

Assignment for the day: If you have wronged someone, give them a call and try to make amends. You may be able to only say that you are sorry, but at least you have tried to make it right.

NOTES:

Gave Blood-Gave Life

John 6:51 I am the living bread which came down from heaven: if any man eat of this bread, he shall live forever: and the bread that I will give is my flesh, which I will give for the life of the world.

While driving down the interstate, I noticed a billboard that read "GIVE BLOOD-GIVE LIFE." As a nurse, I know how true that statement is. Even though I have given blood before, I must confess, I do not donate nearly as often as I could. I've made a personal pledge to myself to do better and donate blood more often. But really, when I read that billboard, the first thing I thought about was "Gave Blood, Gave Life." I thought about how Jesus came to earth, born of the Virgin Mary. God manifested in the flesh so that He could "Give Blood, Give Life" to a lost humanity. I know the Bible says that without the shedding of blood there is no remission of sins and that all have sinned and come short of the glory of God. The Gospels tell about the crucifixion and the horrible death Jesus went through for lost humanity. It was by shedding His blood and becoming the supreme sacrifice that He made eternal life available to all!

My prayer for you today: Dear Lord, I pray for all caregivers reading this little devotion. If they have not already accepted You as their personal Savior and do not have the hope of eternal life, I pray that You show them it can be theirs. Remind them You said in Your Word that You came so we may have life and have it more abundantly. Not just eternal life but a better life here on earth as well. May they know that You can make a way when there seems no way, that You can speak peace into any situation, and that You can give hope when all seems hopeless!

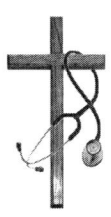

Assignment for the day: If you have not done it lately, make a genuine effort to donate blood over the next few weeks.

NOTES:

Good Report

Philippians 4:8   …whatsoever things are of good report…think on these things.

When I was in RN school, I found the study of mental health to be very interesting. During a lecture on behavior, we found that many believe it is much more productive to focus on good behavior and positive actions. Whether it is in children, teenagers, or adults, praising good behavior gets better results than focusing on bad behavior and actions. As we learned this, my thought was, "You know that is scripture!" Because Philippians 4:8 says, "Finally brethren, whatsoever things are true, whatsoever things are honest, whatsoever things are just, whatsoever things are pure, whatsoever things are lovely, whatsoever things are of good report; if there be any virtue, and if there be any praise, think on these things." I suppose that we all must have good qualities and bad qualities. However, I have found that it is so much easier to look for the good things than focusing on the bad things in people's lives. If you know a nurse, nursing assistant, or any other co-worker that you find really getting on your nerves, why don't you try to focus on three good habits they may have? Once you see the things "of good report" you may find that they do not get on your nerves quite as bad!

My prayer for you today: Dear Lord, I pray for all caregivers today as they do their jobs. Help them that they may look for the best in their co-workers and associates. Help them to remember Your Word and to try their best to focus on whatsoever things are of a good report!

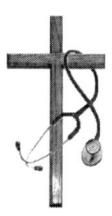

Assignment for the day: If you have a co-worker that gets on your nerves, try to find three (or maybe just one!) good habit she has and compliment her on it.

NOTES:

Guardian Angel

Psalm 34:7 The angel of the Lord encampeth round about them that fear him, and delivereth them.

Some nursing homes have a program called "Guardian Angel" and when new residents are admitted, a department head is appointed to them for their first few months of stay. The department head will visit them a few times a week to make sure they are adjusting to the changes in their environment. The residents usually develop a bond with their "guardian angel" and the transition from home to nursing home is much easier for them. Family members are always glad to hear that their loved ones have a "guardian angel" looking out for them.

In fact, we all would probably like to feel that we have a guardian angel looking after us, helping us, and keeping us from danger. Actually, we really do have one! The above scripture says, "The angel of the Lord encampeth around those that fear God and delivers them." I believe there have been many times a guardian angel has protected me from harm. Numerous times I have been driving and after looking in the rear view mirror to see that it was clear to change lanes, I would change lanes only to see afterwards that a car was right behind me. Other times I have pulled out onto a street and then looked in my rear view mirror and wondered, "Where did that car come from?" I promise I am a safe driver! Once I was leaving the house and happened to remember that I had forgotten to pray for the day. Knowing that I still had a few minutes and that it always means a better day when I can begin it with prayer, I decided to take those few extra minutes and spend them in prayer. When I returned back into the kitchen, I saw that I had left on a burner on the stove! Many of you have had the same situations and can tell of times when you knew there must have been someone looking out for you. Could it have been your "Guardian Angel"?

My prayer for you today: Dear Lord, put a "guardian angel" around each nurse today. Thank You for protection and deliverance that come at times when we are never even aware that we are in danger!

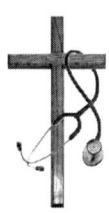

Assignment for the day: If there are people in your life that you know really look out for you, send them a "thinking of you card" and let them know how much you appreciate them.

NOTES:

A Nurse's Prayer

Use these hands, oh Lord, I pray, that You have given me
Open the eyes of those around me that they might be able to see

May all whose fevered brow I touch, receive a touch from You
Use these hands, oh Lord, I pray, in everything I do

The ears of those that cannot hear, the mouths of those than cannot talk
Strengthen the legs of the lame, so they would be able to walk

Each time I see a child sick, its' body wretched with pain
Or see an older person, having to depend upon a cane

When I see a teenager hurt, or a baby with a disease
Something seems to stir within, and I pray, "Use these hands, oh please"

When You called me to work for You, little did I know
That You would give me a burden for the sick, a burden that seems to grow

Without You, Lord, these hands are nothing; but with You, they're everything
When I'm not sure just where to turn, to Your words I cling

I know suffering is not Your will; miracles and healings are not dead
Life and peace and happiness, is why Your blood was shed

I'm only a vessel, Dear God, by myself I'm of no use,
Give me the words to say to others, as I spread the "good news"

You have never let me down; You have answered every prayer
Even when I feel far from You, Your Word says You're still there

Thank You God, for helping this nurse, with everything I do
It may be my hands my patients see, but, Lord, may they feel You

Lord Jesus, guide each step that I take, for it's on You that I depend
Thank You for Your healings, Lord, and use these hands, Amen

Belinda Looney

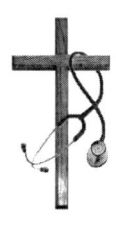

Helping Hands

Isaiah 41:10 Fear thou not; for I am with thee: be not dismayed; for I am thy God: I will strengthen thee; yea, I will help thee…

As I came down the hallway, I watched her leaning forward in her wheelchair. She was reaching for the safety rail and for a second I was afraid she was going to tip forward and fall! Quickly, I gave her wheelchair a gentle push and she was able to grab the rail and do whatever task she had in mind. As I passed by her, I thought of how many times we reach out with helping hands to our residents. Countless times they are unaware they were assisted or helped by someone. Working in a nursing home, I often see the ill effects of Alzheimer's disease, dementia, OBS, etc. Many residents never know of the hands that intervene to prevent them from falling; the hands that gently give PROM; caring hands that give ADL care. Hands that feed; hands that bathe; yes, you might call them "helping hands." Still thinking about this on the drive home, I began to wonder, "How many times has God gently given me a little push in the right direction? How many times have His hands caught me as I was falling? How many times has He assisted me with tasks that were to complicated and difficult for me to perform by myself?" Isaiah 41:10 is one of the most strengthening scriptures for me. When I read it, I am reassured that there is no problem too hard for us if we put our trust and confidence in God to help us! In fact, once I was having a particular hard time after the death of my mother, and I said, "Lord, I need Your help." When I got home, I picked up the newspaper and the Bible scripture for the day was Isaiah 41:10. As I read it, I felt like God was speaking directly to me. He let me know I did not have to be dismayed, He was my God, and He would help me! I stood on that scripture, and true to His Word, God brought me through that situation victorious and stronger than I had ever been!

My prayer for you today: Thank You for being a God who in all Your magnificent splendor will come running to the aid of one of Your children! I pray, Lord, help each nurse that is now going through a difficult time. Bind up any emotional wounds he/she may have and replace any personal turmoil around him/her with peace and tranquility.

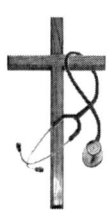

Assignment for the day: Do something for a friend or co-worker today without letting them know you were the one who did it.

NOTES:

If You Don't Use It, You Lose It

I Corinthians 15:58   **Therefore, my beloved brethren, be ye stedfast, unmoveable, always abounding in the work of the Lord, forasmuch as ye know that your labour is not in vain in the Lord.**

As nursing students, we were taught many clinical skills. After becoming nurses, we perfected those skills. However, most of us can agree with what our instructors told us: "If you don't use it, you lose it!" For example, a nurse working on a cardiac floor may become quite proficient reading rhythm strips. But, move her from that area to an area where cardiac monitoring is not routinely done, and over a few years time she possibly will not be quiet as proficient reading them. I remember being so excited when I finally was able to look at a set of ABGs and know how to read them! If I had to read one today, I would have to go dig up the easy formula my preceptor gave me because it's been years since I have even had to look at them. At this time in my nursing career, I am working in a nursing home and mainly do paper work. So the concept of "if you don't use it, you lose it" really concerns me. I was thinking about this the other day, and I feel like the Lord showed me the same is true when it comes to working for Him. There have been times in my Christian life when I have felt that He gave me a burden for a specific area of ministry. As long as I prayed for that area and did what I felt He laid on my heart to do, I kept the burden and could see where He was moving in those areas. I have learned, however, that over time if I slacked off on praying in that area that I would find myself losing the burden. I know there are times when He gives us a burden for something or someone and He removes it. I pray that when He gives me a burden for someone that I will be faithful and not lose the burden until He does remove it!

My prayer for you today: Dear Lord, Help us to be consistent with our prayers and works when You lay a special burden on us. May we not lose that burden until You have truly removed it. Help caregivers to know today that as they do their jobs their labor is not in vain.

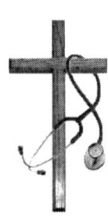

Assignment for the day: Read an article about a disease, medicine or procedure that you have not been exposed to lately.

NOTES:

Is It Really More Blessed to Give Than to Receive?

Acts 20:35   I have shewed you all things, how that so labouring ye ought to support the weak, and to remember the words of the Lord Jesus, how he said, It is more blessed to give than to receive.

Once my daughter asked me if the Bible really says, "It's more blessed to give than to receive." I assured her that it did indeed. Usually, when we quote it, it is around Christmas and we're thinking about gift giving. Or maybe it's at church when we're giving a special offering that we think about it. I know we have all had that "good feeling" that comes from giving that special gift or offering that someone else really appreciated. And we agreed, maybe it is more blessed to give than to receive! However, as I reflect more about this scripture, I begin to consider how it also applies to us as nurses and the many things we "give" to our patients. As a nurse, I have administered or "given" blood numerous times. I am reminded now of how blessed I am to be the one giving the blood instead of the one receiving it! I have "given" many, many pain pills and pain shots over the years to my patients. Now, I have to ask myself, " Am I not more blessed to be the one giving the medicine than the one in pain receiving it?" I think about the many deathly ill patients to whom I have given chemo. One of the major things as nurses that we give our patients is our precious time. Once again, I realize that I am blessed to be able to give my time and listen to someone as he voices his fears over his illness. Because when I think about it, I realize I could be the one "receiving" someone else's time!

Truly it is "more blessed to give than to receive!"

My prayer for you today: Dear Lord, Thank You for blessing nurses with the ability to do their jobs, and may they do them with the compassion so deserving to those who are ill. I pray that You exalt all caregivers today as they give of themselves. As they go about their daily routine, whether it is pain medicine or their precious time they give, may they receive the immense gratification that comes from being in such a fulfilling profession. Moreover, help each nurse today to receive the blessings and promises of Your precious Word in his/her life.

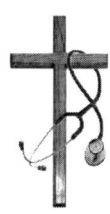

Assignment for the day: Buy lunch for a friend today, or when you go on break with a co-worker buy him/her a soft drink.

NOTES:

Life Is in the Blood

Leviticus 17:11 For the life of the flesh is in the blood: and I have given it to you upon the alter to make an atonement for your souls: for it is the blood that maketh an atonement for the soul.

When I was in LPN school, at times I would just sit in awe as I learned how the Lord made the human body and how it often parallels to the Word of God. While studying the Circulatory System, I felt the Lord showed me this about blood.

FACTS ABOUT YOUR BLOOD:
1. Your blood delivers oxygen (which is essential for life) from the lungs to the cells of the body.
2. Your blood carries away carbon dioxide (a waste product of the cell) from the cells to the lungs where it is exhaled.
3. Your blood delivers nutrients that are absorbed by the small intestine from the food you eat, to the cells of the body.
4. Your white blood cells defend the body against diseases and fight off infection.
5. Without blood there would be no life.

FACTS ABOUT JESUS' BLOOD
1. His blood delivers forgiveness of sins (which is essential for eternal life).
2. His blood carries away hatred, greed, lust, etc. (waste products of sin) from the heart and replaces them with love, joy, and peace.

3. His blood supplies our needs not only for food, shelter, and clothing, but any needs we may have.
4. His blood provides not only healing for our bodies but defends us against the enemy and fights all of our battles.
5. Without His blood there would be no eternal life!

My prayer for you today: Dear Lord, I pray that all caregivers today will reap the benefits of Your precious blood that was shed for them. Let them know that You will fight any battle they may have, and may they feel the love, joy, and peace that comes from knowing You.

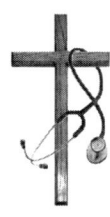

Assignment for the day: If you have not been to church lately, make a special effort to go this Sunday. Also, read about the crucifixion of Christ in the Bible.

NOTES:

Little Ailments

Ephesians 4:11–12   **And he gave some, apostles; and some, prophets; and some, evangelists; and some, pastors and teachers; For the perfecting of the saints, for the work of the ministry, for the edifying of the body of Christ:**

For a little headache, we take two Tylenol. For a little indigestion, we chew on an antacid. For a little trouble with constipation, we increase activity and fluids. Fortunately for us, many small ailments can be taken care of at home without seeking professional help. However, as healthcare professionals, we know if the headache persists, if the indigestion becomes chronic, or if the bowels remain constipated, it could be signs of a more serious problem, and one may need to see his physician. OTC drugs and home treatments are not always enough, and professional help may be needed to prevent serious health complications.

As Christians, there are many small problems and battles we fight on a daily basis. Most of the time with a consistent prayer life we are able to fight these battles and obtain victory without much assistance from others. But just as headaches and indigestion can become so severe they require the help of a professional, as Christians our problems can become severe enough to need the help of a professional! And that is our pastor. The Bible says that God gave pastors and teachers for the perfecting of the saints. He knew that there would be times when we would need advice/instruction from a "professional" in the Gospel.

My prayer for you today: Dear Lord, just as You have given us physicians to help with our physical problems, You have given us pastors to help with our spiritual problems. I pray for all healthcare professionals today that You help them to be attentive to their own physical needs and to seek professional help if needed. As You know, sometimes we are the last ones to seek a doctor for our own needs! I also pray that You help them with any battle they may be fighting spiritually. I pray that they have a pastor in their lives to encourage them and to give that spiritual direction that is so important and beneficial.

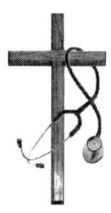

Assignment for the day: Send a card of appreciation to your pastor or someone that you often turn to for help.

NOTES:

Expectations

I want the glamour of the uniform; I'll hold my head up high as I go
Passing all my pills and assessing from head to toe
I want only patients that walk and talk, anything else is forbidden
You'll have to give another nurse the ones that are bedridden
When I walk down the hall, it will be with pride and grace
As confident as I'll be, there won't be a problem that I can't face
Oh, how I want to be a nurse, everything must be just right
With all my time management skills, I'll make it through each night

Now it has been a year, where is my glamour and pride
No one really knows the times, I've wanted to run and hide
Patients can be so demanding, family members even worse
I seem to have forgotten why; I wanted to be a nurse
Sometimes a pill is not enough, patients want much more
How my expectations have changed from what they were before
A person with a disease is also a person too
Looking only at the illness is the worst thing a nurse can do

Now it's been five years, and I'm proud of all my new skills
Sometimes, the last thing I worry about is passing all those pills
Yes, I've made mistakes, each time a lesson learned
I can now give of myself, and expect nothing in return
When a patient comes in the hospital, I no longer see just a disease
I often see a frightened person, so I try to put them at ease
I sit at their bedside and listen, as they reminisce through the years

A closeness soon develops, as we wipe away our tears
When I see a patient coping with their illness at its worse
I remember then——WHY I WANTED TO BE A NURSE

Belinda Looney

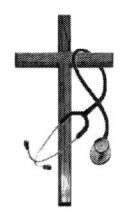

Making It Through

Isaiah 41:6 They helped every one his neighbour; and every one said to his brother, Be of good courage.

Do you ever think about those that helped you make it through nursing school? All of us have those special people, that without their help, we would have never made it! Remember those fellow students that helped cram for tests, prepare for clinicals, and gave the moral support we all needed? After graduating and finally becoming nurses, we find there are still many people who will be helping us "make it through." Some of the nurses that we met while in orientation gave us advice that we still wisely adhere. In fact, I was very fortunate that when I got out of both LPN and RN school I had preceptors that guided me and are my mentors to this very day! May we never forget those special people in our lives. We know that their help, guidance, and encouragement are what helped us "make it through" to become the nurses that we have become!

However, I realize that we still have one more graduation day, and that is when our life here on earth is finished and we have made it to heaven! Just as there were special people to help us make it through nursing school, there are special people helping us "make it through" our every day life as a Christian. Aren't you thankful we have fellow Christians that help us cram for life's tests, prepare for life's clinicals, and give the moral support we all need so much? I suppose I must be a very fortunate person, because just as I had preceptors to teach me to be a good nurse, I have had wonderful "preceptors" to teach me how to be a successful Christian. You know, just as we needed nursing instructors to help us become effective nurses, we need pastors to help us become effective Christians! I thank the Lord for the two wonderful pastors in my life. Surely, when we get to heaven and see Jesus, we will want to thank Him for putting special people in our lives that generously helped us make it through!

My prayer for you today: Dear Lord, I ask that You bless all reading this today. I pray that You give them someone special to encourage and help them on their jobs. More importantly, though, I pray that there is someone in their lives that is encouraging them and helping them to live a Christian life!

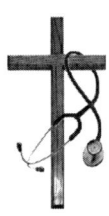

Assignment for the day: If you have nursing students on your floor today, be encouraging to them. Tell them how wonderful and fulfilling a nursing career can be.

NOTES:

Many Members

I Corinthians 12:14–18   For the body is not one member, but many. If the foot shall say, Because I am not the hand, I am not of the body; is it therefore not of the body? And if the ear shall say, Because I am not the eye, I am not of the body; is it therefore not of the body? If the whole body were an eye, where were the hearing? If the whole were hearing, where were the smelling? But now hath God set the members every one of them in the body, as it hath pleased him.

Is that scripture not an awesome lesson on teamwork? It shows us that we're all members of the team and dependent on each other. When everyone works together, it makes the job easier and much more productive resulting in a higher quality of patient care! Just as the eye cannot say unto the hand, "I have no need of thee," or the head to the feet, "I have no need of you," the doctor cannot say to the nurse, nor the nurse to the nursing assistant, "I have no need of you." In fact, behind every great doctor is a great nurse, a great nursing assistant, a great therapist, a great unit clerk, etc. It takes "all" of us, no matter what our position, to ensure that safe, effective care is given to our patients. Everyone is a vital and important member of the team!

My prayer for you today: Dear Lord, Help each doctor, nurse, assistant, therapist, etc. today to realize that he/she is an important part of the healthcare team. Help us all to understand the importance of our individual positions. May we recognize that as a team we are all dependent on one another. Although we have to hold each other accountable for our individual duties, help us to remember that we are a team with an ultimate goal of effective quality care to the patients!

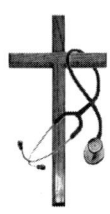

Assignment for the day: Encourage team-work today and let your co-workers (nurses, secretaries, assistants, etc.) know that you appreciate them.

NOTES:

Marrow To Thy Bones

Proverbs 3:7–8 Be not wise in thine own eyes: fear the Lord, and depart from evil. It shall be health to thy navel, and marrow to thy bones.

This is actually the scripture that gave me the inspiration to write this little book of devotions. Since I am a nurse, it caught my attention that Solomon compared the benefits of departing from evil to the marrow of bones. I wondered what he was actually trying to tell us. As I read this, I began to think about the importance of bone marrow and what it does for the body. Knowing that bone marrow produces blood cells and that the Bible says, "Life is in the blood," I believe very simply put, that he is telling us when we fear the Lord and depart from evil it is literally "life" to us! To fear the Lord does not mean that we have to be afraid of Him. It means that we are to be in awe of Him and to reverence Him. God is very adamant in His word about avoiding evil. He does not want us to partake of evil activities and tells us to depart from evil! He knows the danger we put ourselves in when we allow evil to abound in our lives. Many times we unintentionally become involved in things that may be contrary to the Word of God. In our own eyes, we feel like we are strong enough to allow certain things around us that may not be pleasing to Him. We feel we will not become too "involved" and therefore no harm will be done. Unfortunately, before we know it, that small discretionary has gotten us into a huge mess with lots of problems!

My prayer for you today: Dear Lord, You are such an awesome God, and we do reverence You. I pray that You protect all nurses and bless those reading this today with health and safety. Show us the things in our lives that are not pleasing to You and give us the strength to turn from them.

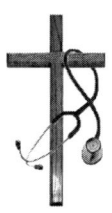

Assignment for the day: If there is an area in your life that the Lord may not be pleased with, ask Him to give you the strength to make the changes you need to make.

NOTES:

Mind Set

Philippians 4:13   I can do all things through Christ which strengtheneth me.

I talked with a physical therapist about success stories in patients requiring therapy. She said one of the main things that make a difference in their recovery is their "mind set." In fact, it was her opinion that far greater results are often obtained when patients enter into the rehab program with a made-up mind to give it their very best! Even though it is a hard struggle and often painful, they know the ultimate goal is well worth it. The Apostle Paul must have had that positive "mind set" when he wrote, "I can do all things through Christ which strengtheneth me." I agree because I have found that most of the time if I really believe I can do something, with the Lord's help, I usually am able to do it! However, many of us will agree that nursing is a field that requires a very positive attitude. I try to begin each day with a positive mind set, but, I must admit, there have been some days when I have left work feeling defeated. Whether it was the frustrations of work in general, or the devastating loss of a patient, I have questioned if I can really do this. Fortunately, I get up the next morning knowing beyond a shadow of a doubt that nursing is for me, and I wouldn't give it up for anything. Because, just like the Apostle Paul, I know that I can do all things through Christ which strengtheneth me!

My prayer for you today: Dear Lord, You know what tasks are before each nurse today. I'm sure some will have a very hard and strenuous day. Give strength to those that are tired and refresh each that has become fatigued. Provide guidance to those that may be questioning their circumstances and encouragement to those that may have become weary! I pray for You to help them to know that You are with them and ready to assist when needed.

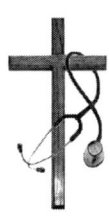

Assignment for the day: If there is something that you have not been able to accomplish, take a fresh look at it, and set a goal to achieve it!

NOTES:

Mission Statement

Matthew 9:37–38   **Then saith he unto his disciples, The harvest truly is plenteous, but the labourers are few; Pray ye therefore the Lord of the harvest, that he will send forth labourers into his harvest.**

Have you ever really read the Mission Statement in the facility where you work? Though different from place to place, they generally have similar goals. Usually the mission or purpose is centered on providing safe effective care, promoting health while maintaining a safe environment, and continuing education to patients as well as the community. When we accept employment at a facility, we also accept the responsibility to ensure that the Mission Statement is carried out. In fact, all the care, all the teaching, and all the precautions taken are a direct reflection of the Mission Statement!

My pastor preaches that the church's Mission Statement should be "The Purpose is Souls!" When you think about it, that's really true, because again, the Mission Statement represents what the organization is all about. In the case of the church, it is Souls! Believing that each person, each soul, will spend eternity either in heaven or hell, makes it all the more important that we help others come to the saving knowledge of Jesus Christ. Just as healthcare providers accept the responsibility of fulfilling the Mission Statement of their facility, as Christians, we are responsible to seeing the church's Mission Statement is fulfilled. I feel that helping someone, a soul, come to the saving knowledge of Jesus Christ is one of the greatest accomplishments as a Christian that I can achieve.

My prayer for you today: Dear Lord, Help us today as we do our jobs. Help us to give safe, effective care to our patients. At the same time, help us to see our patients as souls, and may Your love reflect through us in the care we give. As nurses endeavor to carry out the mission statement of their employer, help them to realize that they are important to You, and You care about any need they may have. If they do not know You as their personal Savior, I pray, Lord, help them come to Your saving knowledge.

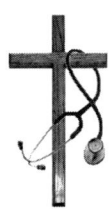

Assignment for the day: Read the Mission Statement in your facility and give yourself a pat on the back for your contribution to it being fulfilled!

NOTES:

No Procedure Is Small...

Philippians 4:6   **Be careful for nothing; but in everything by prayer and supplication with thanksgiving let your requests be made known unto God.**

When I was in RN school, one of my instructors said something that to this day I still find so true! She said, "No procedure is small when it is being done to you or one of your family members." I began to think about all the nursing procedures we do that seem so simple and routine. Just think about all the times you have taken blood pressures or temperatures. How many UA's and sputum specimens have you collected? Important, yes, but all routine for us as nurses! When my husband was once admitted to the hospital, I was reminded of my instructor's words of wisdom. When the nursing assistants would take his temp, I found myself asking, " Has it came down?" When the nurses took his blood pressure I asked, "What was it?" When his lab results came back I inquired, " How were they? What did his UA show?" Yes, very routine procedures, but as a family member they were very important to me. On the spiritual spectrum, I think the same principle can be applied. No prayer request is too small for God! Almost every day we hear about desperate people requesting prayer for impossible situations. Their only hope is that God will intervene for them. With so much tragedy, diseases, and turmoil going on, one is almost hesitant to request prayer for something that seems "small." Lost keys, nagging headaches, minor aches and pains, surely God is too busy with frantic requests to bother with these simple ones! Thankfully, He is not too busy! Because He is our Father and we are His children, even our smallest requests are important to Him. Aren't you glad that nothing is too big or too "small" for God?

My prayer for you today: Dear Lord, I pray that You assure all caregivers today that You are concerned about even the smallest of their needs. Let them know that by prayer and supplication with thanksgiving, they can let any request be made known unto You.

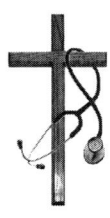

Assignment for the day: Pray about something you may feel is too small to bother God about. See if He doesn't come through for you.

NOTES:

Nurses' Appreciation Week

Jeremiah 3:15   And I will give you pastors according to mine heart, which shall feed you with knowledge and understanding.

Too many times nurses receive the brunt of a patient's frustration over being sick. Unfortunately, many clients leave the nursing facility without ever giving thanks to their healthcare provider. Everyone likes to feel appreciated, and nurses are no exception! So when Nurses' Week rolls around, we all enjoy the small gestures made by others to show thanks for all we do. Whether it's pizza that is ordered for lunch by the docs, fancy cookies delivered by a special carrier, or a "thank you" card from management, we all enjoy the treats. No matter how large or small they are. We love our profession and we did not choose it for the "thank yous," but they sure are appreciated.

Pastors can probably identify with us because there are no doubt many days they go without anyone showing them gratitude or appreciation! They give so much of themselves. Holidays, vacations, special time with family, all occasions are prone to be interrupted by a desperate phone call from a saint in need. My mother passed away on Christmas Day, and guess who left his family and came to the hospital to comfort my family? My pastor. When my son-in-law was in a fatal car wreck, who do you think was with us all through the hospital stay? My pastor. When I stand before God and hear Him say, "Well done, my good and faithful servant," who am I going to be able to thank for giving me the preached Word that I needed to make it? My pastor. Many do not know that October is actually Pastors' Appreciation Month. At our local assembly, we celebrate all month by doing things for our pastor. Pastors love their "profession" and did not choose it for the "thank yous," but, just like caregivers, they sure feel good when they are appreciated!

My prayer for you today: Dear Lord, Just as You have given pastors to feed Your people with knowledge and understanding, You have given nurses to care for the sick with compassion and understanding. Help those that are receiving care today to be a little more sensitive and thankful to those that are giving care to them. May each caregiver feel appreciated and know how important he/she is to the healing of the sick!

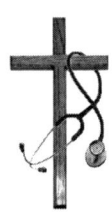

Assignment for the day: Let your supervisor or manager know how much you appreciate him/her.

NOTES:

Personal God

Isaiah 41:10   …for I am thy God…

As a rule, I know that I should not share my personal life with my patients. I must admit, though, that I have had some patients that by the time they were discharged I felt like I had known them, and their families, for a long time. But on the most part, I try to keep a professional relationship and not become too personal with them. Aren't you glad that is not how we have to be with God? I would like to tell you a little incident that happened to me at work one day. It helped me realize I truly serve a "personal God."

While I was in the elevator on my way to the lab, for some reason, I began to think about my mother. She had died several years earlier. I guess after someone dies you start thinking about all the things you never talked about. Well, for some odd reason I had the thought, " I'll never know about Mom's wedding to her first husband, George." She didn't talk about him very much and certainly didn't talk about her wedding to him. I don't even know why I was thinking about it that day. I had resolved that I would never know about it. I want you to know, that when I got off the elevator and went to the lab, there was a woman there that I had seen before but hadn't really talked to much. She looked straight at me and said, "I want to tell you about your mother's wedding to George Luther!" Come to find out, she knew my mom and her family when she was growing up. She told me all about her wedding, her dress, and about the people at the wedding. When I left the lab, I was almost dumbfounded! Not because I had heard about the wedding, I had wondered about, but what amazed me was that I finally realized that I serve a personal God! He knows all about my wants and desires. He knows me personally!

No one will ever convince me that it was just a coincidence that THAT lady was in the lab and wanted to tell me THAT particular story at THAT particular time! No, you see, I serve a personal God who cares about even the smallest details in my life. Not only did this help me spiritually, it also helped me to help my patients because as a nurse I see lots of people in pain and despair. I see them at some of their most heartbreaking times. Since that day in the lab, I have been able to tell my patients that they serve a personal God. He knows exactly who they are and what is going on with them! He is your personal God, too. He knows where you are and what's going on in your life. Are we not a blessed people?

My prayer for you today: Dear Lord, I pray for all caregivers today that You show them that You are indeed a personal God and that You care about every aspect of their lives. Help them to get the revelation that although there are millions of other people with problems and needs, You care about each one of us individually! Your Word tells us that You are no respecter of persons. Reassure each one reading this today that he/she is special and important to You. Remind each one that if he/she was the only sinner in the world, that You love him/her enough that You would have still suffered Calvary for that one individual! You truly are a personal God.

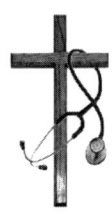

Assignment for the day: Pray to God about one area in your life you feel you can't talk to anyone else about. Remember that nothing it too embarrassing or too shameful to tell Him.

NOTES:

Puzzles, Pieces, and Pictures

Romans 8:28   **And we know that all things work together for good to them that love God, to them who are the called according to his purpose.**

Many times when patients seek medical help, they expect the doctor to know rather quickly what is "wrong with them." He is expected to have all the answers to their questions because, after all, he is the doctor! Realistically, when the doctor sees the patient for the very first time, the client actually presents as a big "puzzle." It is only after gathering vital information such as history, lab results, x-rays, etc. that all the "pieces" of the puzzle are put together. The doctor is then, hopefully, able to make a diagnosis and prescribe the right treatment completing the "picture."

I once heard a sermon entitled "Puzzles, Pieces, and Pictures." When you think about it, that's the way our lives are. When you are born, you are presented as the puzzle. Throughout your life, there will be many pieces added and some taken away. Most will make sense, but there will be some that you do not understand. The majority of pieces of the puzzle will bring joy and laughter. Some will bring sorrow and pain. There will be mystery pieces, embarrassing pieces, and pieces that you question. As your life progresses and all the pieces are put together, the whole picture evolves, and the result is "you"!

My prayer for you today: Dear Lord, You know all about us. You know all the embarrassing details, the things that have brought us laughter, and the things that have brought us pain. Help those reading this today to be reassured that even though they may be going through something they do not understand, You are here to help them and to bring the "pieces" together.

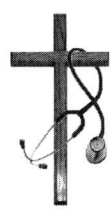

Assignment for the day: Tell at least two doctors that you work with today how much you appreciate them.

NOTES:

Rejoicing and Weeping

Romans 12:15   Rejoice with them that do rejoice, and weep with them that weep.

"Rejoice with them that do rejoice, and weep with them that weep." In the nursing field, this really rings true! It is so awesome to share in the joy of families waiting those last few hours for the birth of their special baby. Grandparents, aunts, uncles, godparents, and friends are everywhere. The waiting room often overflows with people "rejoicing" at this momentous time. When that little baby boy with all ten fingers and toes intact is placed in the nursery for all to see, it brings a smile to everyone! Being a med/surg nurse for several years, I was often one of the "rejoicers" when family members got that call from the OR "She made it through the operation fine and is going to be okay." Though busy doing our jobs, we are often included in the "waiting period" and therefore included in the rejoicing when good news comes.

Unfortunately, it is not always good news we have to share. "She didn't make it through the surgery," "He is eaten up in CA and there's nothing more we can do," are words dreaded by all. Even though we are professionally trained not to get emotionally involved with our patients, it is still often heart breaking. Most of us will admit we have had our times when we wept with those that wept. Whether it was comforting the young mother that was left alone to raise her three-year-old son; reassuring the eighty-five-year-old man now left to live his last few years alone; or consoling the parents horrified that their teen-age daughter was in a fatal car accident; yes, there are times we weep with those that weep.

My prayer for you today: Dear Lord, You know what lies ahead of those giving care today, and I pray that there be much more reason for rejoicing than weeping. Also, may there be reason for much rejoicing in the personal lives of each caregiver today.

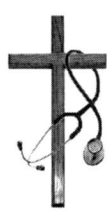

Assignment for the day: Try to be a little extra sensitive today. If you encounter someone rejoicing, congratulate them; if someone is weeping, comfort them.

NOTES:

Specialty Areas

Proverbs 3:6   **In all thy ways acknowledge him, and he shall direct thy paths.**

We had a missionary from Africa visit our church. As he told us about life in Africa, I must confess I was glad it was he instead of me going over there to minister to lost souls. I began to think about the many different areas of the ministry. There are foreign missionaries that go to foreign countries, home missionaries that build churches here in the USA, evangelists that preach revivals all over the country, youth ministers that minister to the youth, and then, of course, there are pastors that minister to individual congregations. No doubt, there are numerous other areas of ministry. I am sure they all have spent many hours in prayer about their particular ministry. One thing they all have in common is their desire to see souls saved and to see that the Word of God is preached all over the world. Just as there are many different areas of ministry with all one common goal, there are many different areas of nursing with one common goal. That goal is helping the sick. No doubt, many of us asked for divine intervention when deciding what area to choose for nursing careers. You may be working in surgery assisting the surgeon as he performs life-threatening operations, or be a med/surg nurse who takes care of the patient after surgery. Perhaps your specialty is intensive care, cardiac rehab, day surgery, management, emergency, geriatrics, dialysis, chemotherapy, or discharge planner. No matter what the area, again, all the caregivers have one common goal and that is to see that safe effective care is given to each patient assigned to their care. Just as the minister knows that every person is a soul that must be reached, the nurse knows that each client is a patient that must be cared for safely.

My prayer for you today: Dear Lord, Thank You for the promise to direct our paths. Help all caregivers today as they go to the special area You have given them to work in. Help them to provide safe effective care to each client, and may that client receive healing to his body through the hands of Your servants. For those that now have major decisions to make, I pray that You help them to remember if they acknowledge You that You will indeed direct their paths!

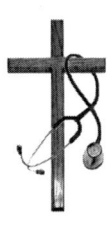

Assignment for the day: Read Proverbs chapter 3

NOTES:

The Cure

In loving memory of my sister, Joan Sanford,
who lost her battle with breast cancer

Acts 2:37–39   **Now when they heard this, they were pricked in their heart, and said unto Peter and to the rest of the apostles, Men and brethren, what shall we do? Then Peter said unto them, Repent, and be baptized everyone of you in the name of Jesus Christ for the remission of sins, and ye shall receive the gift of the Holy Ghost. For the promise is unto you, and to your children, and to all that are afar off, even as many as the Lord our God shall call.**

Do you think there will ever be a cure for cancer? Will scientists and researchers ever find a cure for Alzheimer's disease? Will diabetes only be "controlled" and never cured? Will those suffering from ALS be cured in this generation? How many thousands of people will die of AIDS before a cure is found?

Is there a cure for hatred? Is there a cure for greed and lust? Is there a cure for whatever it is that causes someone to feel he can take the life of another? Is there a cure for lying, stealing, and cheating? Is there a cure for sin?

We hope and pray that someday a cure will be found for devastating diseases like cancer, Alzheimer's, AIDS and ALS. Many of us have been tragically affected in someway by one or more of these fatal diseases. But for the question, "Is there a cure for sin?" the answer is "Yes!" We read in the book of Acts that on the day of Pentecost, Peter preached a great sermon to a multitude of people. In fact, Scripture says it pricked their hearts and they asked what should they do. Peter told them to "repent, be baptized in the name of Jesus Christ for the remission of sin," and they would receive the gift of the Holy Ghost. That was over 2000 years ago, and the cure for sin is still the same! The Bible tells us that all have sinned and come short of the glory of God. Aren't you thankful we have an advocate in Jesus Christ and that He gave us a "cure" for sin?

My prayer for you today: Dear Lord, May a cure soon be found for the devastating diseases that invade the lives of people today. Help those that have either directly or indirectly been affected by them. Facilitate researchers and scientists as they search for these coveted cures. Also, help each nurse today to know that although the cure for sin is over two centuries old, it is still as effective and plentifully available to all who desire it! For this we are eternally grateful.

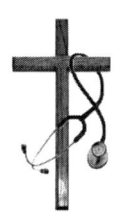

Assignment for the day: If you have not had a physical or a mammogram in the last few years, CALL TODAY, and make an appointment.

NOTES:

The Good Samaritan

Luke 10:34 …and bound up his wounds, pouring in oil and wine, and set him on his own beast, and brought him to an inn, and took care of him.

I think we are all familiar with the parable of the Good Samaritan in the Bible. Basically, it tells us the story about a man who fell among thieves. They wounded him, robbed him, and left him for dead. A priest and a Levite passed by him and did not offer to help. Then we read of the Good Samaritan that saw him, had compassion on him, and bound up his wounds. He took the man to an inn and paid the expenses to take care of him while he recovered. Jesus asked the question, "Which of the three was neighbor unto him that fell among thieves?" He then instructs us to go and do likewise.

    I would like to tell you a story of a patient I once had. This woman had made some bad choices and had gotten into a very bad life style. She had become involved with drugs and alcohol. They, like the thieves in the parable above, wounded her, robbed her, and left her for dead. The drugs wounded her body making her heart go into congestive heart failure. They robbed her of the love and security of her family. They left her without hope of a better life. I'm sure the enemy just knew he had her in the palm of his hands; but you see Jesus had other plans! The woman's sisters and father traveled out of state to go get her and bring her home. The Good Samaritan in this story is a doctor at the local hospital. He heard of how the woman had been robbed and wounded by the effects of drugs and alcohol. He knew she had no money to pay him for his services. Yet, he told the sisters to bring her to his office, and a whole series of events were started to put her on the road to recovery!

Today, that woman is living a life she never dreamed she could have. She accepted the Lord as her Savior and attends her local church faithfully. Thank the Lord for people who are willing to be Good Samaritans!

My prayer for you today: Dear Lord, I pray as all caregivers perform their work today, let them do it with the spirit of the Good Samaritan. Help them to have compassion for their patients and be reminded of Your gentleness. Likewise, may they in turn be blessed and receive the same compassion and gentleness from others.

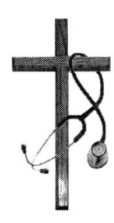

Assignment for the day: Read Luke chapter 10

NOTES:

The Great Physician

Mark 5:25–29 **And a certain woman, which had an issue of blood twelve years, And had suffered many things of many physicians, and had spent all that she had, and was nothing bettered, but rather grew worse, When she had heard of Jesus, came in the press behind, and touched his garment. For she said, If I may touch but his clothes, I shall be whole. And straightway the fountain of her blood was dried up; and she felt in her body that she was healed of that plague.**

Without the accomplishments of many great scientists and physicians, the world would not be as we know it today! Alexander Fleming's accidental discovery of penicillin and Louis Pasteur's invention of pasteurization were gigantic accomplishments. From Christian Bernard's performance of the world's first human heart transplant to the works of international recognized cardiovascular surgeons, hope has been given to heart patients all over the world. Whether from the local county hospitals or large facilities like the William Mayo Clinic or St. Jude Children's Research Hospital, great physicians have ultimately touched millions of people. Yes, great men of medicine have altered our lives and the lives of future generations! Did you know Jesus was known as the "Great Physician"? In the three short years of His earthly ministry, lepers were cleansed, the lame walked, and blinded eyes were opened, all on His command. Just as Jesus had compassion on those that were sick over 2000 years ago, He still has it for the sick and diseased today! Although God still does miraculous healings, He often uses medicine/surgery, by the hands of earthly physicians, to bring healing to those that are sick. From general practitioners to brain surgeons, thank the Lord for great physicians today!

My prayer for you today: Dear Lord, I pray for the physical needs of those reading this today. As nurses, we are so busy taking care of the needs of our patients and families; we often neglect ourselves. Help each nurse today to be conscientious of her own health needs and to see her doctor if she has a health problem and has been "putting it off." Thank You for the great physicians that help so many people today and thank You for being the Great Physician!

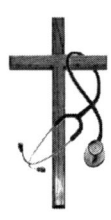

Assignment for the day: If you have not called to get an appointment for your mammogram or physical yet, CALL TODAY.

NOTES:

Thank God for the Blood

John 19:33–34   **But when they came to Jesus, and saw that he was dead already, they brake not his legs: But one of the soldiers with a spear pierced his side, and forthwith came there out blood and water.**

From the 8-year-old hemophiliac who needs repeated transfusions of factor VIII or IX concentrate to stay alive: THANK GOD FOR THE BLOOD!

From the 23-year-old trauma victim who needed multiple units of PRBC before stabilizing: THANK GOD FOR THE BLOOD!

From the 28-year-old renal patient admitted to the hospital with an hct of 18 and discharged with one of 34: THANK GOD FOR THE BLOOD!

From the 30-year-old father of three who has just been healed of pancreatic cancer: THANK GOD FOR THE BLOOD!

From the 40-year-old crack cocaine addict who just had a miraculous change in his life by coming to the delivering knowledge of Jesus Christ: THANK GOD FOR THE BLOOD!

From the 90-year-old faithful saint who came to the saving knowledge of Jesus Christ seventy years ago and is now on her deathbed ready to enter into Glory: THANK GOD FOR THE BLOOD!

My prayer for you today: Dear Lord, thank You for giving mankind medical knowledge that is used to save lives, and thank You for medical miracles that still amaze us all! More importantly, thank You for Your precious blood that was shed for our healing and salvation. I pray a special blessing for every healthcare professional today that truly knows the blessing of "The Blood." I pray for those reading this today that are in difficult situations and may have given up all hope. Whether it is a physical need or a spiritual need, I pray, Lord, that You intervene for them and perform a miracle in their lives. May they truly see why Your blood was shed.

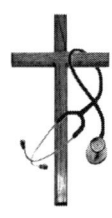

Assignment for the day: You have a two-fold assignment for today. First, read Isaiah 53:5-8. Also, don't forget to donate blood at the next blood drive!

NOTES:

Wages

Romans 6:23   **For the wages of sin is death; but the gift of God is eternal life through Jesus Christ our Lord.**

Nursing can be a hectic vocation, and many days nurses feel like they do not get paid nearly enough money! But for me, on the most part, it has been very rewarding financially. While in nursing school in 1991, I worked at BMH in Memphis as a nursing assistant. I started there making more per hour than I ever had. With minimum wage being three dollars and thirty-five cents per hour, I was really on my way up making five dollars and fifty cents an hour! After graduating LPN school, I started my nursing career making eight dollars and twenty- three cents an hour. Of course, the wages have gotten much better, and like I said, nursing has been good to me financially. However, I believe a rewarding nursing career is actually just one of the benefits of my main vocation. You see, as a Christian my ultimate "job" is to live every day of my life to the best of my ability! It is recognizing that when I fall short I have a Savior who is there to lead and guide me. It's trying to see the good in everyone and everything. It is helping others and sharing my blessings. My Pastor once asked a high school graduating class, "Are you going to work for "change" or are you going to work for "change?" If I meet someone during the course of my shift that needs up lifting due to his circumstances, my desire is that in some small way I will have brought change into his life. Maybe it was only by an understanding smile or an encouraging word; nonetheless, for a few moments he knew someone cared!

My prayer for you today: Dear Lord, I pray that You help all caregivers today. Bless them financially, physically, and more importantly spiritually. Help them to reap the benefits of their skillful vocation, and encourage them to accept the challenge to not just work for "change" but to work for change.

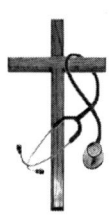

Assignment for the day: Give a special offering this Sunday or send someone a card with a few dollars in it.

NOTES:

Epilogue:

For many of us, deciding to go to nursing school was an easy decision! Some dreamed of being nurses while they were just little girls. In their imaginary world, their dolls became patients as they cooled their brows from make believe fevers or wrapped their broken limbs with gauze and tape. Dad's white T-shirt was their favorite uniform. For others, like myself, it was a decision made later in life. As a family, we had to sit down and "count the cost." There were many things to consider, and as a family we agreed we were willing to make the adjustments. My daughters had attended a Christian school for several years, and that year we were able to do the custodial work for their tuition. Because I would have to quit work and we would only have one income, we moved into a small trailer we owned. My husband, Bobby, and my two daughters, Holli and Jennifer, were wonderful during this time of adjustment. I know it was a hard year for them, but they were great and gave me the moral support that made it all much easier, and for that I am so thankful. I love and appreciate them all so much. However, there was one area with which I would not compromise, and that was my relationship with God. Because of the encouragement and strength that comes from attending church faithfully, I made a personal promise to myself before starting school that I would not miss church to study for a test. I believe God honored that decision because I actually did pretty well grade wise for someone who had been out of school for seventeen years! My final devotion is called "Counting the Cost."

Counting the cost. What does that mean? Does it mean deciding if you have enough money to pay for something? Does it mean considering the consequences of decisions you make? Does it mean willing to suffer pain and humiliation, even death, to give life to someone else?

Counting the Cost

Luke 14:28   For which of you, intending to build a tower, sitteth not down first, and counteth the cost, whether he have sufficient to finish it?

I Timothy 3:16   And without controversy great is the mystery of godliness: God was manifest in the flesh, justified in the Spirit, seen of angels, preached unto the Gentiles, believed on in the world, received up into glory.

The little girl looked at the pile of coins in one hand and then at the white plastic corsage in the other hand. Smiling, she was flooded with thoughts of homemade sugar cookies, ice cube trays filled with frozen grape Kool-Aid, and other treats that her mom always had waiting for her sisters and her after school. Very simple things to some people, but they seem to always make the little girl and her four sisters seem so special. "Still," she thought, "it has taken a long time for me to save up all these coins!" It seemed like it took forever for all of them to jingle out of the tin can she used for a piggy bank. She knew it would take her a long time to save up that much money again. "What should I do?" she pondered.

"Buy the corsage for Mom? If I do, it will cost me all of my money. Or should I just keep saving all of it? It's not like it is her birthday or anything. If I keep saving until Christmas, there's no telling how much I will have! Hmmnn, what should I do?"

The beautiful smile on her mother's face when she was presented with the small white corsage let the little girl know she had made the right decision. Those coins were a small price to pay for a memory that would last throughout the little girl's lifetime!

Married only six years, that seemed more like twenty, the young couple sat facing each other wondering what they should do. They were so sure when they had gotten married that it would be for life. But here they sat now, feeling like strangers, not even friends anymore. They were both still young. If they divorced now they would each probably find love again. Maybe then it would be for life. She would be free to follow her dreams and he would be free to follow his. But what would the cost be and would they be willing to pay it?

Their little girls lay sleeping, not aware of the turmoil around them. The young couple looked down at them, the only "good" thing from their marriage. They were four-year-old identical twins. The pride and joy of not only the couple, but also of both their families, too! Gorgeous, adorable, precious, all words too inadequate to describe them in their parents' eyes. He knew that if they got a divorce he would still get to see his girls. But would weekends and holidays be enough? Those were his girls and he didn't know if he could take the chance of them having a stepfather someday. She knew that he would always support his daughters. But she also knew they would need much more than financial support. She didn't want them to have just a weekend father, someone good for gifts, but possibly wouldn't be there when he was really needed. Was the happiness and security of those little girls too high of a price to pay for the freedom and happiness they believed would come from a divorce?

When the couple renewed their wedding vows on their twenty-fifth wedding anniversary, they looked into the eyes of those little girls, now beautiful young women. They were both so thankful they had been willing to pay the price that kept their family together!

God Almighty, the Creator of the universe, the Giver of life, looked down from Heaven's throne to lost humanity. He knew when He created man that someday this day would come. It was time for the supreme sacrifice to be made for His creation, mankind. Surely, He had to be aware of the price He would have to pay to save men from their sins! What would the cost be? Could even God Almighty pay such a price to save man? Would He be willing to be manifested in the flesh, be denied by His closest followers, be spit upon and slapped by His very creation? Could He withstand the thorns, as they would tear into His scalp, the nails, as they would be hammered into His flesh? Surely He knew about the beating He would receive! Would He be able to withstand it as the coat of flesh is torn from His body? Could the Creator withstand such treatment from His creation? Certainly that would be too high of a price to pay, even for the Creator of the universe! Even if He did pay it, would His heart be able to withstand the fact that many of His creation will still deny Him and not accept salvation even after such a supreme sacrifice? But how else could mankind be saved? How could healing be purchased if God wasn't willing to pay the cost? How could words like hope, joy, faith, peace, and love ever be known to His creation if He weren't willing to pay the cost?

More than 2000 years later, God Almighty smiled down from Heaven's throne and saw His creation, men and women. Although there were still many who had not yet accepted Him as Lord and Savior, He saw millions as they were praising Him, worshiping Him and repenting of their sins. Thank You, Lord, for paying the cost for our salvation.

My prayer for you today: Dear Lord, thank You for all caregivers who have read this little book of devotions. I pray that it has brought encouragement and inspiration to them. I pray that they realize You are a personal God who knows and cares about every one of them. I pray that they recognize how important they are to Your service and that it is through their hands and words that You often minister to people who are sick. I continue to pray Your blessings on all Healthcare Professionals! Protect us and protect our patients. In Jesus name we pray. Amen.

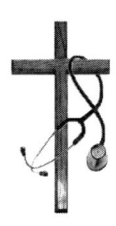

I have written this little book of devotions in loving memory of my mom, Polly Richardson Grigsby. Although she passed away before I became a nurse, I know she would be so proud of me today! My prayer is that her sweet and kind spirit will live on through my daughters and me.

"MY SAVIOUR"
May 13, 1982

GOD IS MY LOVE, MY WAY OF LIFE
HE HELPS ME EACH DAY, THROUGH MY STRIFE

WITHOUT HIM, I'M NOT REALLY LIVING
EACH DAY IS FULL OF HIS GIVING

HE'S IN MY HEART, EVERYDAY
HE KEEPS ME GOING ON MY WAY

WHEN I NEED HIM, HE'S ALWAYS THERE
HE HEARS AND ANSWERS EVERY PRAYER

WHEN I DIE AND TAKE MY REST
I'LL BE IN THE ARMS OF THE ONE
THAT I LOVE BEST

POLLY RICHARDSON GRIGSBY
1930–1989

About the Author

Jenny Morris was born in Snyder, Texas, and when she was one year old, her parents moved to Arkansas where she has lived ever since. She trained at Mid-South VoTech (Now Mid-South Community College) in West Memphis, Arkansas, and East Arkansas Community College in Forrest City, Arkansas. She began LPN school at the age of 35 and RN school at the age of 40 believing as many do that "it's never too late to go back to school!" Jenny is the wife of Bobby Morris and the proud mother of twin daughters, Holli and Jennifer. She is the very proud grandmother or "Nanna" to one grandson, Drew Griffin. Jenny attends church at the First United Pentecostal Church in West Memphis, Arkansas, where she is very active in the Ladies' Ministry and the Jail Ministry. As well as being a wife, a mother, a grandmother, and a nurse she is a Christian and loves the Lord with all of her heart! Her desire is that all will hear of the "Good News" and come to the saving knowledge of Jesus Christ! You may contact her at jennymorrn@sbcglobal.net

ISBN 1-41205008-1

Made in United States
North Haven, CT
07 June 2022